*This manual was written to assist doctors and (
in the treatment of their patients, and more impo
help their patients help themselves.*

— **Michael**

SELF-HELP MANUAL

Managing Back Pain

by
Michael S. Melnik M.S., O.T.R.
Robin Saunders M.S., P.T.
H. Duane Saunders M.S., P.T.

Published by
The Saunders Group, Inc.
4250 Norex Drive
Chaska, MN 55318-3047

612-368-9214 or 800-654-8357
Fax: 800-375-1119

Table of Contents

INTRODUCTION............................3
BACK CARE BASICS.......................4
ACTIVITIES OF DAILY LIVING...........6
Sleeping.................................6
Getting into/out of Bed...................8
Bathing..................................9
Bathroom Activities.....................10
Dressing................................11
Sitting.................................12
Standing................................13
Making the Bed..........................14
Getting into/out of Car.................14
Driving.................................15
Laundry.................................16
Kitchen Activities......................16
Child Care..............................18
Shopping................................19

Vacuuming...............................21
Mowing..................................21
Car Maintenance.........................22
Shoveling...............................23
Home Maintenance........................24
Sexual Activities.......................24
Recreational Activities.................24
LIFTING.................................25
Golfer's Lift...........................26
Deep Squat Lift.........................26
Diagonal Lift...........................27
Modified Diagonal Lift..................27
One Knee Lift...........................28
Partial Squat Lift......................29
Straight Leg Lift.......................29
SUMMARY.................................30

ISBN Number 0-9616461-6-0

copyright 1989
H. Duane Saunders

Managing Back Pain

A Self Help Guide To Participation In Daily Activities For Back Pain Sufferers

Many people with back pain unknowingly aggravate their conditions by participating in stressful activities of daily living during the healing process. This manual is designed to prevent this continued aggravation by teaching you how to safely perform many common activities while you are recovering from back pain.

When people experience back pain, they often either stop participating in all activities or continue to perform activities despite a significant increase in pain. Both extremes are usually inappropriate. *While it is important to rest following an injury, it is also necessary to participate in some form of physical activity.* The recovery process is based on a balance between the appropriate levels of activity and rest.

This manual is put together in a way that will allow you to progress in your activities of daily living as your condition improves. Recovery generally falls into three categories: ACUTE, SUB-ACUTE, and STABLE. Each stage requires a different approach in the number and types of activities performed.

Acute: During the acute, or early phase of your recovery you may be experiencing substantial pain/discomfort. The goal at this time is to minimize the stress to your back during the basic activities of daily living, such as sleeping, bathing, dressing, going to the bathroom and eating. *Unnecessary activities should be avoided at this time.*

Sub-Acute: During this phase the intensity of your back pain has diminished and your doctor or therapist may have instructed you to increase your activity level. The goal is to become more active while minimizing your symptoms. It is the combination of these two that will maximize the speed of your recovery. *It is important to remember that even during the sub-acute stage you must choose your activities carefully, and choices for new activities should be discussed with your therapist or doctor.*

Stable: During this phase it becomes very important to return to an active lifestyle with the goal being to prevent further episodes of back pain. The manner in which you perform your work and activities of daily living has a direct influence on the condition of your back. *Do not take the absence of symptoms to mean that you can return to performing tasks in the same stressful manner as you did before your back pain occurred.*

Back Care Basics

Several principles of proper back care are detailed on the following pages. The main principles which will be addressed are the following:

1. **Maintain the normal curves of the back.**
2. **Plan your movements ahead of time.**
3. **Ask for assistance when appropriate.**
4. **Do not remain in one position for extended periods of time.**
5. **Maintain a wide, stable base while standing and lifting.**
6. **Pivot your feet, don't twist your back.**
7. **Keep your stomach muscles firm while lifting and participating in daily activities.**
8. **Keep items close to the body when lifting or carrying.**
9. **Lift with your legs, not with your back.**
10. **When in doubt — ask your therapist or doctor.**

If you understand the above principles and implement them into your daily activities, you will decrease the stress on your back and speed the healing process.

This manual will help you understand the types of movements which can continue to irritate your condition and show you alternate ways to perform many activities of daily living without increasing your pain or making your problem worse.

One of the keys to having a healthy back is maintaining the curves of the spine in a *balanced position.* If one of the curves becomes either flattened or excessive (too much curve), the balance and mobility of the spine may be altered and undue stress is placed on the back.

Movements and positions in this manual are identified as those which increase the stress on your back (Unbalanced) and those which reduce the stress on your back (Balanced).

BALANCE IS THE KEY

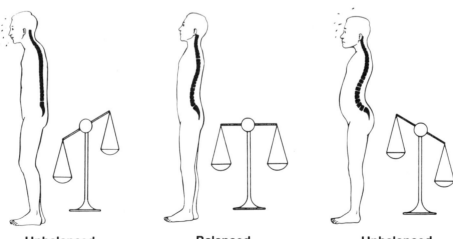

| Unbalanced | Balanced | Unbalanced |

It is important to remember that most back problems are not the result of a single injury. Even though pain is often felt suddenly, such as during a twist or lift, the problem is almost always due to a combination of several factors.

Most Back Disorders Are the Result Of ...

1. **Poor Posture**

2. **Faulty Body Mechanics**

3. **Stressful Living and Working Habits**

4. **Loss of Flexibility**

5. **General Decline of Physical Fitness**

With few exceptions, back problems are the result of months or even years of stress to the spine. These factors accumulate throughout one's lifetime during both work and home activities. *Managing Back Pain* is designed to help you protect your back from continued aggravation. The rest of this manual describes specific techniques for performing a variety of daily tasks.

Not all techniques may be appropriate for you. Try them, modify them and consult with your therapist or doctor to find what works best for you.

You will notice that there is quite a range of activities included in this manual. *Many of the activities presented are NOT appropriate for the earlier stages of recovery.* They are included to help you prevent a recurrence of your symptoms once your condition has stabilized and you have returned to an active lifestyle.

Remember: It is going to take time for you to be able to incorporate these new movement patterns into your daily life. The more you practice these techniques, the more natural they will become.

Activities of Daily Living

Sleeping/Resting

Even if you are experiencing a severe episode of back pain, many activities are unavoidable. Bathing, dressing and sleeping are relatively simple tasks, but may aggravate your back problem if performed incorrectly. In all of these activities, the back must be kept in a balanced position.

We spend one-third of our lives in bed, yet we often neglect to consider the effect this has on our backs.

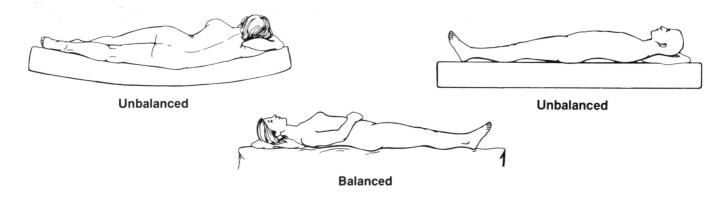

Unbalanced   Unbalanced

Balanced

A mattress should be firm enough to prevent you from sinking, yet soft enough to conform to the normal curves of the body. Waterbeds are acceptable, especially if they are waveless or tubular, and if they are filled adequately.

When choosing a bed, consider that a king or queen size mattress allows more movement during the night. This reduces stress on the joints and muscles and can reduce morning stiffness.

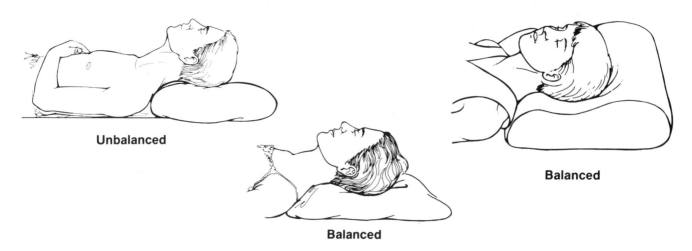

Unbalanced   Balanced

Balanced

The pillow should support your neck and allow it to rest in a balanced position. A feather or fiber pillow is best because it conforms to the shape or your neck better than foam. Some foam pillows which are specially contoured to support the neck are acceptable.

Sleeping/Resting

It is important that you sleep in positions that promote the healing process. While you may have limited control over the postures you move into while sleeping, you are able to choose certain positions when resting or preparing for sleep.

If you are waking in the morning with increased symptoms the following changes may help:

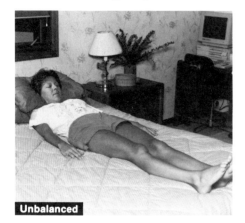
Unbalanced

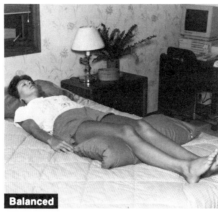
Balanced

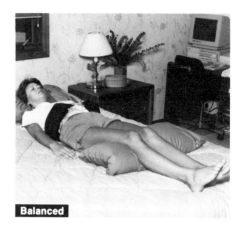
Balanced

1. Sleeping/Resting On Your Back

Avoid the use of pillows which place your neck in an unbalanced position. A small pillow under your knees may increase your comfort; a large pillow is not generally recommended. Night rolls, such as the one pictured, are designed to keep your low back in a balanced position while you sleep.

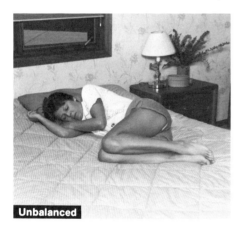
Unbalanced

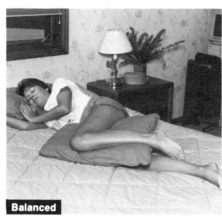
Balanced

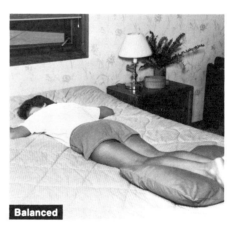
Balanced

2. Sleeping/Resting On Your Side

It is generally not recommended to bring both knees in towards your chest when sleeping or resting on your side. Although this position may temporarily feel comfortable, it is not a balanced position for your back. Keep your lowermost leg nearly straight and bend your top leg. A pillow placed between your legs can increase your comfort.

3. Sleeping/Resting On Your Stomach

Sleeping on your stomach is not necessarily a bad idea. This is especially true if you have a good, firm mattress that doesn't sag. Usually a pillow for your head is not recommended while sleeping in this position, but placing a pillow under your feet to bend the knees and ankles a bit may increase your comfort.

Getting in and out of Bed

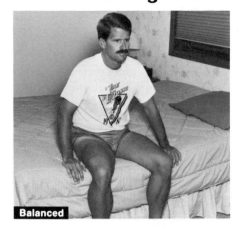
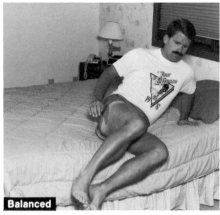
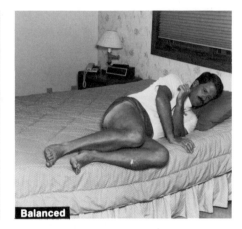

1. To get into bed, sit on the edge of the bed, then lower your upper body sideways, using your arm for support. At the same time that you are lowering your upper body, bring your legs and feet up onto the bed. If you have someone who can assist you, he or she can help by slowly raising your legs as you lower your upper body to the bed. To get out of bed this process is reversed.

Twisting and bending can often be minimized during this task by firming up your stomach muscles before you begin to move. Twisting can also be reduced by using only the arm closest to the bed for support, eliminating the need to reach across your body.

Before attempting to stand, scoot as close as possible to the edge of the bed and place your feet on the floor. Use a night stand for support if available, or push with your hands against your thighs. Keep your head up and your back in a balanced position. *Remember that your muscles have cooled and tightened during the night. Use care and move slowly when getting out of bed in the morning.*

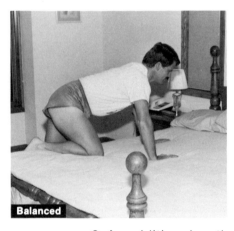
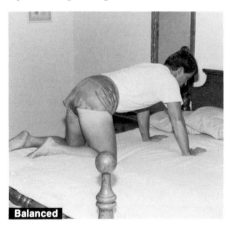
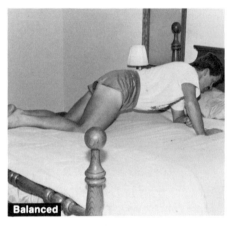

2. An additional method for getting into bed is to support your upper body on the edge of the bed. Slowly crawl onto the bed while you keep your back in a balanced position. Once you are on all fours you can lower yourself with your arms. To get out of bed this process is reversed.

Note: Many people suffering from back pain choose to sleep or rest on the couch. The couch does not offer you the support of your bed and encourages an unbalanced posture. In addition, changing positions during the night can reduce morning stiffness, and these important movements are severely limited when sleeping on the couch.

Bathing

Showers are usually better than baths because the balanced position of your back is easier to maintain while standing. It is also safer to get into and out of a shower than a tub.

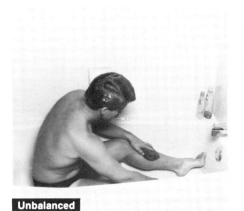

Unbalanced

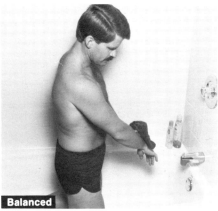

Balanced

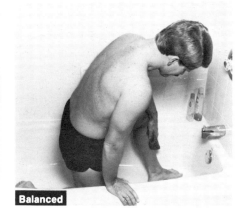

Balanced

If you don't have a shower, and sitting causes increased pain, you can take a bath in a kneeling position. A small towel can be placed under your knees to increase your comfort. When you must bend forward, be sure to support the weight of your upper body on the edge of the tub.

Place a bath mat in the tub to reduce the chance of slipping. Losing your balance, even if you don't fall, can aggravate an existing back problem. Ask for assistance getting into and out of the tub when necessary.

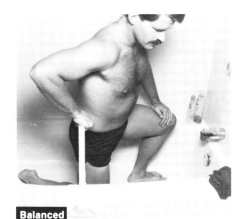

Balanced

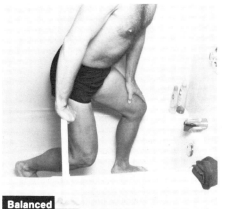

Balanced

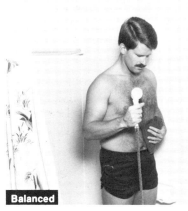

Balanced

For those who have long-term or recurring problems, installing a grab bar can increase both the ease and safety of getting into and out of the tub or shower. If you don't have a shower, you may wish to invest in a shower hose which will allow you to stand.

Keep items within easy reach. If you shower, install a rack between waist and shoulder height for your personal articles.

Dressing

While you are experiencing acute back pain, you should allow yourself extra time in the morning to dress. Hurrying often causes one to neglect the use of proper body mechanics. Also, the following tips may help:

Wear slip-on shoes to eliminate the need to bend forward. Items such as tight slacks, socks and nylons are often difficult to put on and may need to be avoided during the acute stage. Wear loose fitting clothing, such as sweatpants, to increase the ease of dressing.

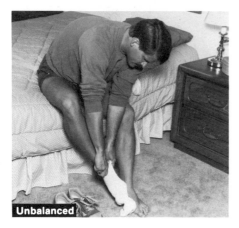 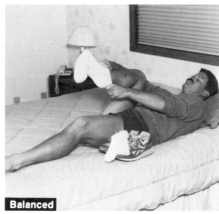 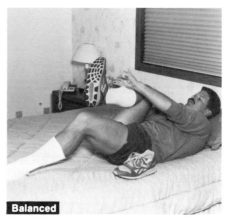

Avoid getting dressed while sitting at the edge of the bed or standing with your back forward bent. Put on underwear, slacks, nylons and socks while lying down.

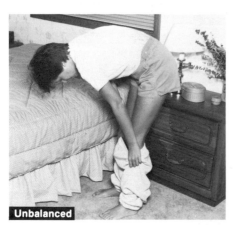 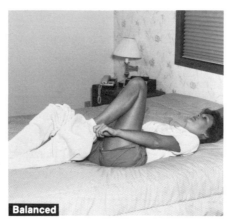 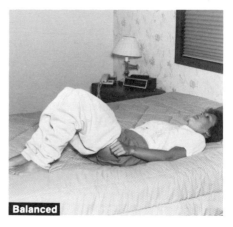

Keep your back flat on the bed and pull your clothing up as far as you can. Next, roll onto your side and stand up (see page 8). You can then finish dressing in the standing position.

Remember that undressing can be as stressful to your back as dressing. The methods described above will work for both situations.

Bathroom Activities

As mentioned earlier, forward bending places increased stress on the structures in the back and neck.

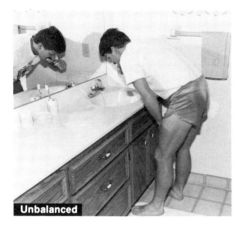
Unbalanced

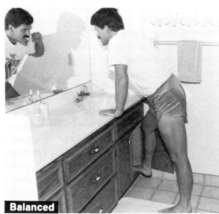
Balanced

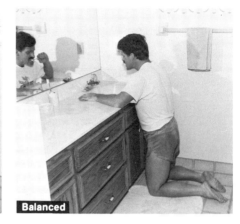
Balanced

If you are going to work over the bathroom sink, place one hand on the counter to support your weight and bend at the hips, not the back. Elevate one foot and keep your head up and your back in a balanced position.

You can also try performing some of your sink activities in the kneeling position to reduce the temptation to bend forward. Use the counter for support when you come to standing.

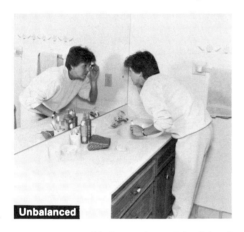
Unbalanced

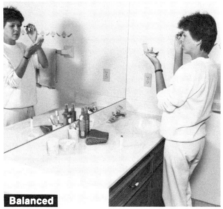
Balanced

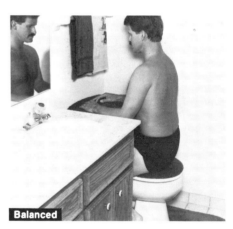
Balanced

Using a hand-held mirror eliminates the need to bend over the sink.

During an acute episode of back pain you can minimize stress when using the toilet by facing the back of the toilet. This will prevent you from bending forward and will provide you with support when you come to standing.

Sitting Posture

It is important to realize that sitting, particularly with your back in an unbalanced position, can place more stress on your back than standing or lying down, and therefore should be minimized as much as possible during the acute stage of injury.

Occasionally, people with back pain feel that a slumped or forward bent position is comfortable. The comfort is misleading, however, because it places a continual stress on many structures of the back and neck, thus delaying the healing process.

Rules of Sitting

1. Don't sit too long (15 – 20 minutes maximum). Sitting while listening to music or watching television, particulary on a couch that does not provide proper support, can place additional stress on your back and should be avoided during the early stages of recovery.

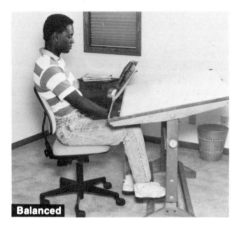
Balanced

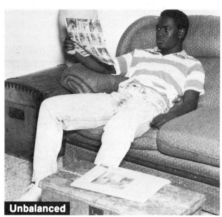
Unbalanced

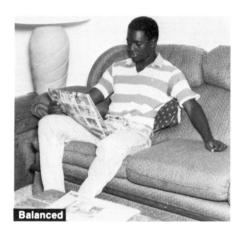
Balanced

2. Sit in a chair or couch that provides proper support for your low back. A good chair will help you maintain the normal curves of your spine. If your chair or couch does not provide proper support for your low back, a small pillow or rolled towel can be used.

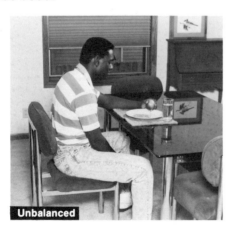
Unbalanced

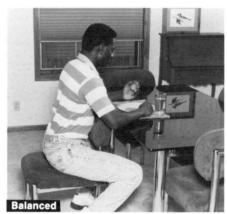
Balanced

3. Do not sit in a slumped position with your head resting in front of your shoulders. You can reduce the stress of sitting by turning a chair around backwards and straddling the seat. This encourages you to sit up straight and the back of the chair provides support for your upper body.

4. If sitting and working, place your materials in a position which allows you to sit up straight. A copy stand to elevate your work and an adjustable height chair and table are helpful and commercially available.

Rules of Sitting *(continued)*

5. Both feet should be supported on the floor or foot rest.

6. If sitting at a desk or table, try to sit in a position which allows you to rest your forearms on the table without needing to bend over. This allows your arms to support some of your upper body weight and discourages you from bending forward.

7. Do not sit in deep or low furniture. This may feel comfortable temporarily, but your spine is placed in an unbalanced position. It is also difficult to rise from this type of furniture without forward bending.

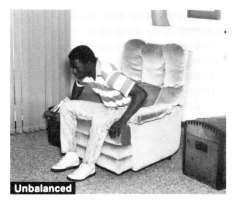
Unbalanced

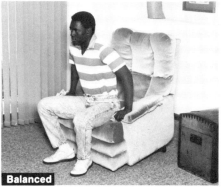
Balanced

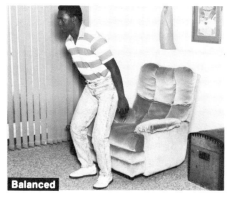
Balanced

It is important in all situations to move to the edge of the chair or couch before you attempt to stand. Push off with your arms when beginning to stand. If support is not available, try reaching your hands above your head as you prepare to stand. This movement will encourage you to keep your head up and your back in a balanced position while beginning to stand.

Standing Posture

Slumped shoulders and a forward head posture place stress on your back and neck.

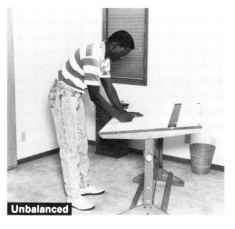
Unbalanced

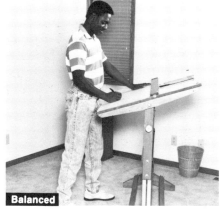
Balanced

Keep your head over your shoulders, your shoulders over your hips, and keep a comfortable/wide base of support with your knees slightly bent. This will allow the muscles of your legs to absorb more weight and reduce the stress to your low back. Adjust your work height so that you maintain a balanced posture.

Keep your stomach muscles firm while standing. This reduces the weight bearing pressure on your back. Wearing good supportive soft-soled shoes also reduces the stress to your back. Avoid wearing hard-soled or high-heeled shoes.

Making the Bed

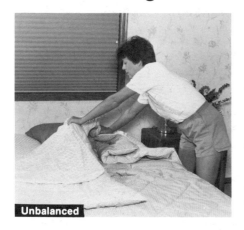 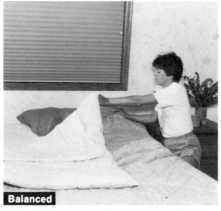 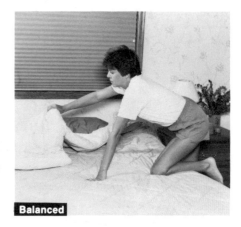

When making the bed, do not stand on one side and reach. The temptation to bend forward can be reduced by kneeling or climbing onto the bed. This will encourage you to keep your back in a balanced position. If you are going to perform the task while standing, walk around the bed to complete the far side.

Getting into a Car

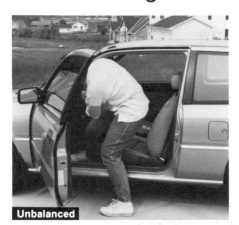 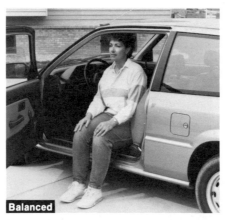 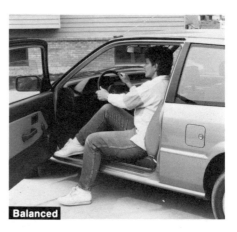

Sit down in the car facing out the door. Slowly bend your legs and bring them into the car as you rotate your head and shoulders toward the front. If you will be driving, use the steering wheel for support. Move your shoulders and hips together and turn your body as a unit. To get out, reverse this process.

Driving or Riding in a Car

While driving or riding in a car or truck, it is important to maintain a balanced posture.

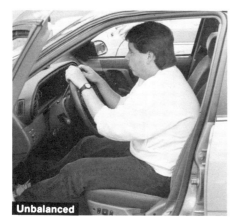
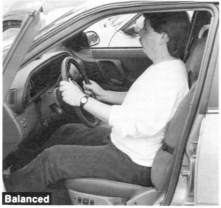
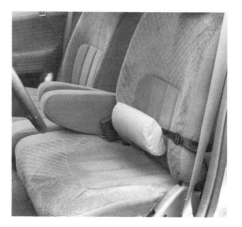

The seat back should be tilted slightly backward. This position places the least amount of stress on the structures of your back. Slide the seat forward so you do not have to reach for the pedals or steering wheel. Grasping the steering wheel toward the bottom reduces the need to bend forward while driving.

A lumbar pillow or rolled towel helps maintain the normal curves in your back. Ask your therapist or doctor for assistance when determining the type of support which is most appropriate for you. Use cruise control, if available, to allow for more frequent changes of position.

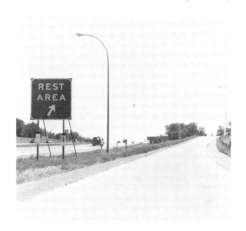
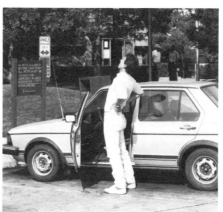
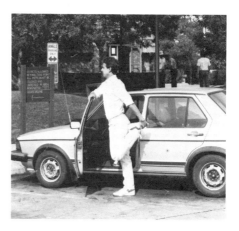

If you will be in the car for extended periods of time, you should get out of the car and stretch every 30 to 45 minutes to relieve the stress of prolonged sitting. Change positions frequently to reduce the stress on your back.

Extended periods of driving should be avoided during the acute and sub-acute stages.

Laundry

Keep loads small and manageable. Several small loads will place less stress on your back than one or two large ones.

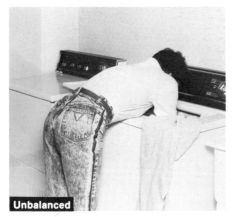
Unbalanced

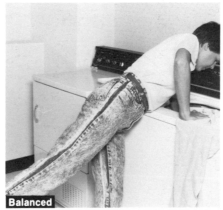
Balanced

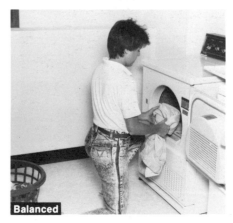
Balanced

Avoid bending forward into the machines. For top loading machines, utilize the golfer's lift or straight leg lift to avoid bending your back (see pages 26 and 29). Do not try to handle large bundles of clothes, particularly if they are wet. When loading or unloading a front-loading washer or dryer, drop to one knee to avoid any forward bending and twisting. Use support when coming to standing.

Kitchen Activities

It is very important to avoid tasks or positions which do not allow a balanced posture. Take a few seconds to approach each task in a way which will minimize the stress to your back.

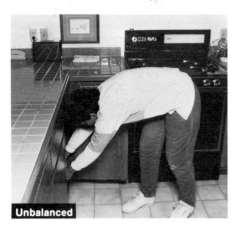
Unbalanced

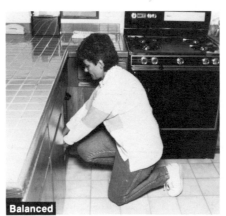
Balanced

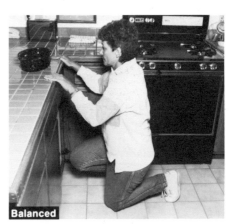
Balanced

Arrange commonly used items between waist and shoulder height to reduce the need to bend over. If you need to reach something from a lower level, drop down onto one knee, grab the object, put the object on the counter and then use the support of a table, chair or counter to assist you while you come to standing. This support will help you maintain the normal curves in your spine. If you do not have support available, place your hands on your thighs and push off with your arms.

Kitchen Activities *(continued)*

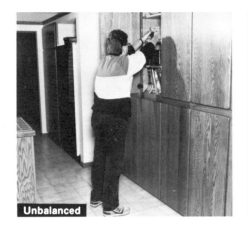 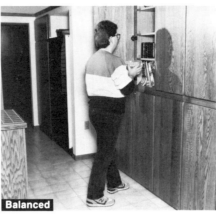 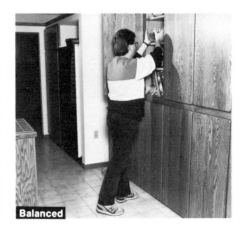

When placing items overhead, place one foot slightly ahead of the other, facing the shelf. Keep your head up and your back in a balanced position.

Shift your weight from the back foot onto the front foot as you move the item towards the shelf. This allows you to keep the load close to your center of gravity and reduces the stress on your back, neck and shoulders.

This weight shift is reversed when removing items from the shelf.

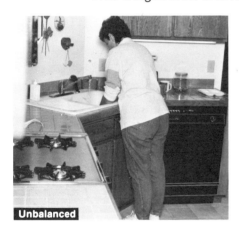 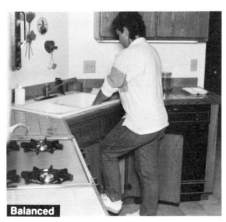 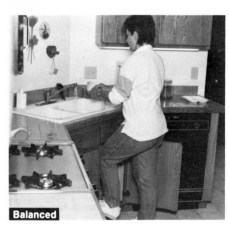

Avoid bending over your work. When standing at the kitchen sink for extended periods of time, open a lower cabinet door and place one foot on the bottom shelf. This helps to keep your back in a balanced position. You can also hold dishes up and close to you while washing them. This encourages you to maintain an upright posture.

Try sliding heavy dishes rather than lifting them. You may want to invest in a serving cart to move heavier items around the kitchen.

Kitchen Activities *(continued)*

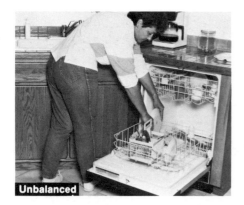
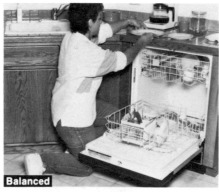
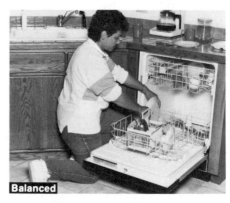

To load the dishwasher, place the rinsed dishes on the counter near the dishwasher. Go to one knee and load the dishwasher from this position. This helps you avoid prolonged or repetitive forward bending and twisting movements. Reverse the process to unload the dishwasher. Use support when you come to standing.

Child care

You must take special care when handling children if you are experiencing back pain. Sudden movements can increase your pain and interfere with your ability to handle the child safely. This places both you and the child at increased risk.

Avoid changing your child on the floor if you have a changing table or elevated work surface available. When bending over the dressing table or crib, bend at the hips rather than the waist and keep your back in a balanced position. Some cribs have sides that fold down which eliminate the need to bend forward and reach. If you do not have this option, the straight leg lift (see page 29) will allow you to pick up your child while keeping your back in a balanced position.

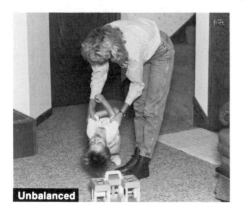
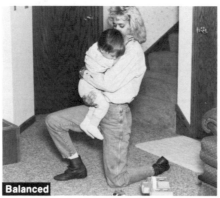
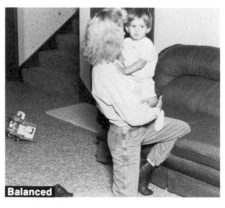

Limit the amount of lifting you do. When you must lift a child from the floor, use one of the methods described in the "lifting" section. The one-knee lift is often the most effective and safe (see page 28). The child should be as close to your body as possible before beginning the lift. Keep your back in a balanced position.

If the child is old enough, have him stand up or sit on a chair or couch prior to picking him up. You can then slide him onto your knee or use a partial squat lift (see page 29). This decreases the distance you must lift and eliminates the need to bend forward.

Avoid carrying a child on one hip for extended periods of time. While it may free up a hand, this unbalanced position places excess stress on the back.

18

Shopping

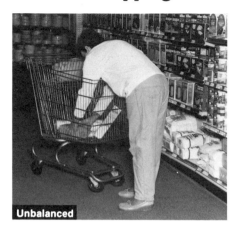 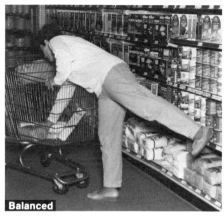 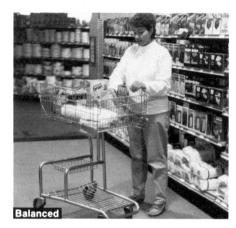

Do not bend forward at the waist to place items into your cart. The golfer's lift (see page 26) allows you to place or reach items with minimal stress to your back. Some stores provide shallow carts which eliminate the need to forward bend.

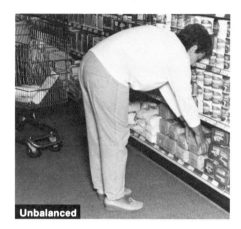 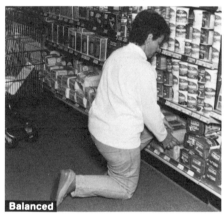 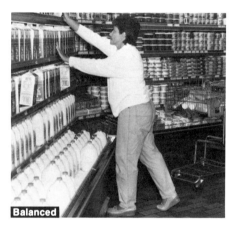

When retrieving items from a lower level, go to a one knee position. This will allow you to keep your back in a balanced position. Use support when you come to a standing position.

When items are located overhead, get as close to the item as possible and use one hand for support.

Shopping *(continued)*

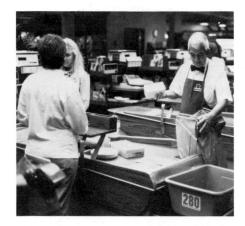
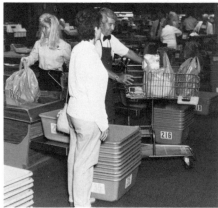
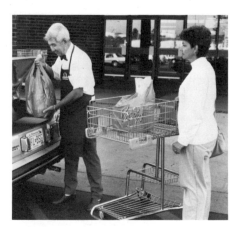

Request assistance in both bagging and carry out. Several small loads will be easier to manage than a few heavy ones.

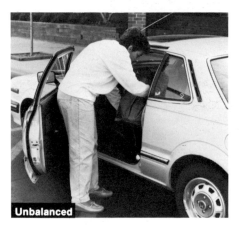
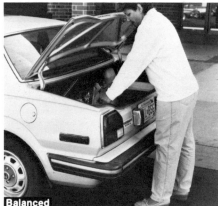
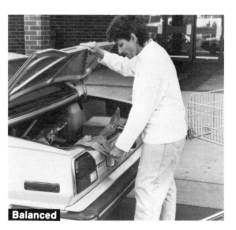

Place groceries in the rear of the trunk, not in the back seat of the car. They are easier to handle from the trunk. When placing or removing the bags, get right up against the back of the car and bend forward at the hips and not the waist. Keep your back in a balanced position.

Often groceries fall over during transit, forcing you to bend forward and reach deep into the trunk when unloading. This can be eliminated by requesting plastic bags with handles which are available in some stores. Set them at the rear of the trunk with the handles sticking outside. When you close the trunk, the handles will be held in place, preventing the bags from spilling. When you get home, the bags can easily be unloaded with minimal bending.

NOTE: *Participation in the following activities (vacuuming, car maintenance, mowing and shoveling) is not recommended during the early stages of recovery.* These activities are presented to offer methods for preventing a recurrence of your symptoms once your condition has stabilized.

Sweeping/Vacuuming

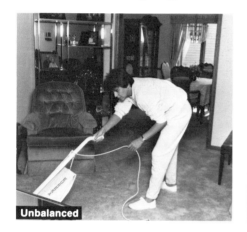 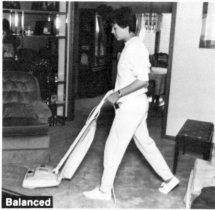 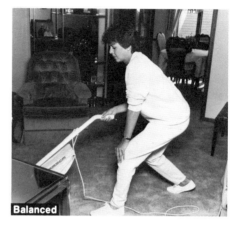

Perform the task as if the vacuum or broom were attached to your body. Move your feet and legs rather than reaching or bending forward. Avoid twisting. If you must vacuum or sweep under a table or chair, bend at your hips and knees and keep your back in a balanced position.

Mowing

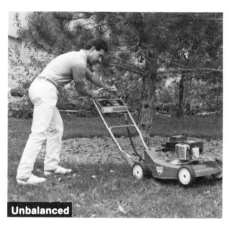 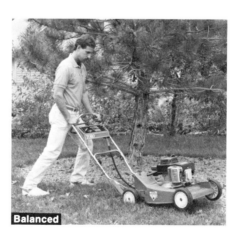 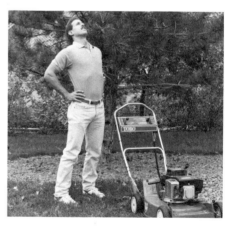

When mowing, avoid twisting your back. Pivot your feet and always face your shoulders and hips in the direction the mower is heading. This is particularly critical when mowing around trees/shrubs or on inclined surfaces. Be sure to keep your stomach muscles firm, your head up and your back in a balanced position. Take frequent stretching breaks to reduce the stress on your back.

Car Maintenance

As mentioned earlier, it is important to determine whether or not this activity is appropriate for your level of recovery.

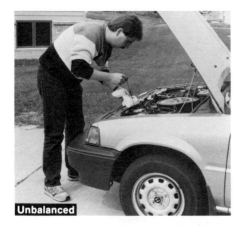 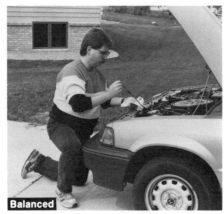 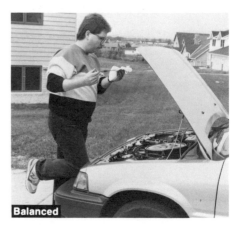

Bending over at the waist should be avoided. When possible, kneel or squat to get closer to your work.

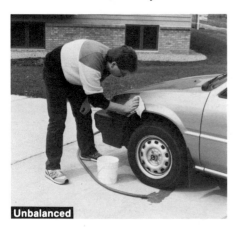 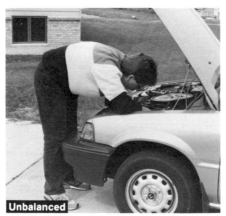 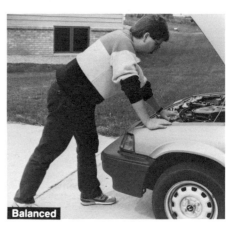

When you must work at lower levels, keep the weight of your upper body supported with one arm and bend at the hips, not the waist.

As with all activities, change positions frequently and stretch.

Shoveling

Shoveling can be a stressful activity for the back even for a person who is not experiencing back pain. *It is not recommended that you participate in this activity until your condition is stable.*

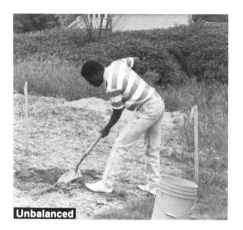
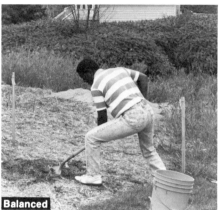
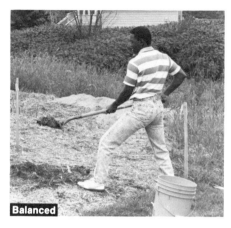

When shoveling, bend at the hips and knees, not the waist. Keep the shovel close to your body and use your legs to lift the load, not your back.

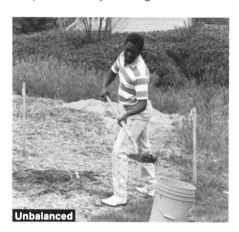
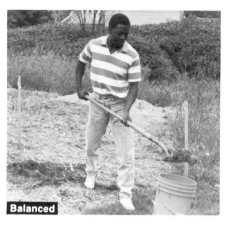

Do not stand in one spot and throw the load. This encourages you to twist your back. Instead, turn and step to keep your hips and shoulders moving in the same direction. Remember to keep the load close to your center of gravity.

Home Maintenance Tasks

1. As in any task, first evaluate the necessity. *Is this activity appropriate for your level of recovery?*

2. Kneel when performing work at lower levels. Do not bend over at the waist.

3. Do not remain in any one position for extended periods of time; take frequent breaks. Learn to pace yourself.

4. Maintain the balanced position of your back during all tasks.

5. Avoid situations that may result in any rapid jerking motions. These types of motions can aggravate an existing back problem.

Sporting Activities

As has been repeated throughout this manual, *it is important that you discuss participation in potentially stressful activities with your doctor or therapist.* They can work with you to determine whether or not a particular activity is appropriate for your condition. In general, sporting activities which require forward bending, rapid change of direction, or twisting of the back can be especially stressful and should be restricted or approached with caution while you are experiencing back pain.

Recreational activities, such as fishing, can add stress to your back because they may cause you to maintain unbalanced postures for extended periods of time. *The rules for sitting and standing posture at home and work apply equally to recreational activities.*

Sexual Activities

Back pain can limit your physical abilities, thus limiting your sexual activity. It is important to realize that you and your partner can participate in a sensual, loving relationship even when experiencing the frustration of back pain.

Generally, you and your partner must experiment with activities and positions which support the spine in a balanced position. The book, *Sex and Back Pain,* by Lauren Hebert, RPT is an excellent reference for participating in comfortable sex when experiencing back pain.

Lifting

Before lifting, evaluate the necessity and recognize your limitations. The appropriateness of particular lifts should be discussed with your doctor or therapist. During the early stages of recovery, it may be more appropriate to simply leave an item on the floor and allow someone else to pick it up.

You may have received certain restrictions from your doctor regarding the amount of weight you can safely lift. *A safe lift must not only address the amount of weight being lifted, but also the manner in which it is lifted.*

Contrary to popular belief, the back muscles are not meant to perform lifting activities. The main purpose of the back muscles is to work in combination with the stomach muscles to help you maintain a balanced posture while you lift. The lift itself should be performed using the larger muscles of your legs and buttocks, not your back.

It is difficult (and impractical) to eliminate all lifting tasks from your daily activities. While this may be necessary during the earliest stages of recovery, you will begin to lift more as your condition improves. It is important that you incorporate the principles listed below when performing any type of lift.

Rules for Lifting

1. **Plan your lifts and remove obstacles from your path.**
2. **Test the weight of a load before attempting to lift it.**
3. **Ask for assistance when necessary.**
4. **Keep your back in a balanced position throughout the lift.**
5. **Use your legs for lifting as much as possible.**
6. **When lifting, keep the load as close to your body as possible.**
7. **Tighten your stomach muscles while lifting. Don't hold your breath.**
8. **Pivot your feet instead of twisting your back if you need to turn while lifting.**
9. **Replace quick/jerking movements with smooth ones.**
10. **Minimize reaching and bending.**

A variety of different lifting methods will now be described. While remembering the principles outlined above, choose the lifting method which is most appropriate for your situation. *You may want to practice these lifts with your therapist or doctor to insure that you are performing the techniques correctly.*

For lifting very light items, try using a broom handle with tape on the end. This will work for pens, pencils, paper clips, etc. . . and will eliminate the need for you to bend over.

The Golfer's Lift

This lift is most appropriate for light objects and is often easier for individuals with decreased leg strength or painful knees.

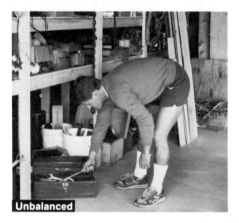 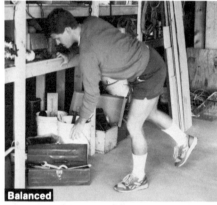 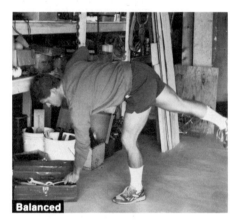

Bend at the hips while raising one leg behind you. While holding onto a solid object for support, pick up the item with your free hand. Lifting one leg helps to keep your back in a balanced position. To return to the upright position, push off with your arm while lowering your leg. This lift is only appropriate for light items which can be lifted with one hand.

The Deep Squat Lift

This lift is most appropriate for small, lightweight items, and when you have support available to assist you as you come to a standing position.

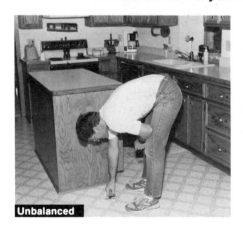 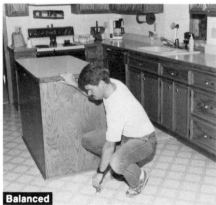 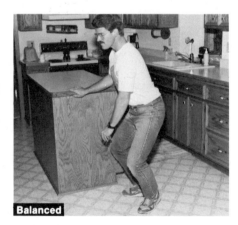

Be sure to keep the item close to your body and your back in a balanced position throughout the lift. If you do not have support available, push off with one hand on your thigh as you begin to stand. This lift should be avoided by people with knee problems. An additional method for lifting light items from the floor is the one knee lift (see page 28).

The Diagonal Lift

The diagonal lift is used when lifting moderately heavy items from floor level.

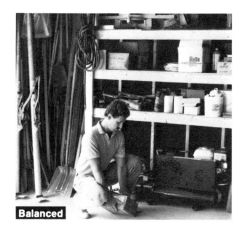
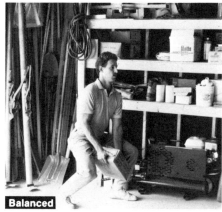
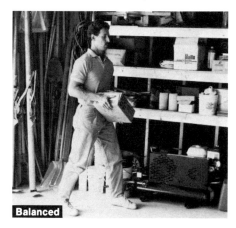

This lift is performed as shown with your legs shoulder width apart and one foot slightly in front of the other. This will provide you with a wide base of support. The item should be moved as close to your body as possible before initiating the lift. The load should be located between your legs, not in front of your knees.

The key to this technique is keeping your back in a balanced position, keeping the weight close to your body and using the strength of the legs to lift. As you stand, the head should rise first, with no movement in your back. *If you are lifting incorrectly, your hips will rise first and force the weight to be lifted by your back.*

The Modified Diagonal Lift

The modified diagonal lift is used to lift larger items or items which are elevated one to two feet off of the floor or items which have handles.

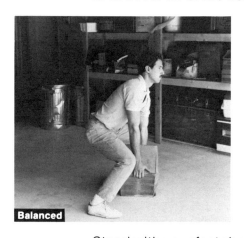
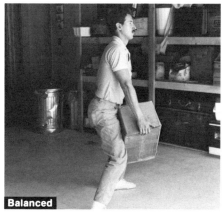
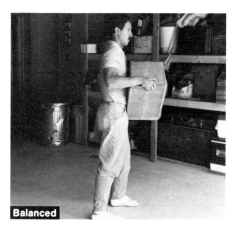

Stand with your feet shoulder width apart and one foot ahead of the other. Your legs should be bent into a half squat position and your body positioned slightly over the load. You can get closer to the load by bending at the hips. No bending at the waist should take place. With your head and shoulders up complete the lift. Keep the item close to your body.

The One Knee Lift

This technique is good for certain bulky or awkward items which are located on the ground.

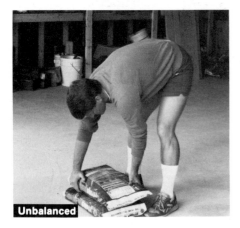 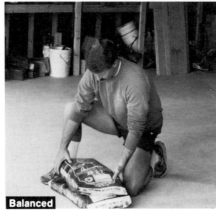 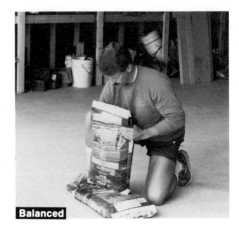

The one knee lift allows you to bring items close to your body before you begin to lift.

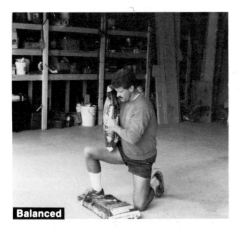 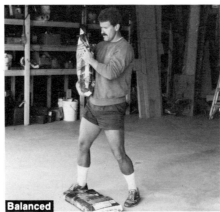 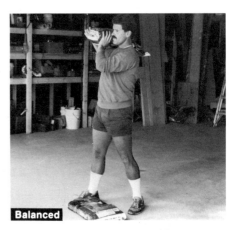

Kneel beside the object to be lifted and bring the object up onto the opposite thigh as shown.

Keep your head and shoulders up as you begin the lift. This will help you keep your back in a balanced position. When carrying an item for an extended distance, carry it on your shoulder. This keeps one hand free for opening doors and allows you to see obstacles that may be in your path.

The Partial Squat Lift

This technique reduces the stress on both the back and the knees.

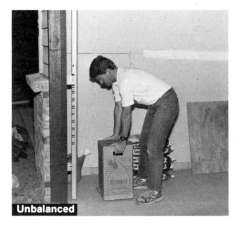
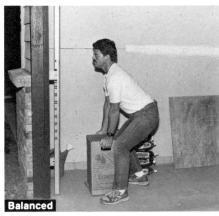
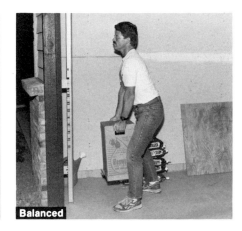

This lift is especially helpful for lifting items which are near knee height. Bending at the knees and hips helps to avoid forward bending at the waist. You should stand with your feet approximately shoulder width apart and one foot slightly ahead of the other. This will give you a wide base of support and allow you to bring the load close to your body before lifting.

If an item can be lifted with one hand (ie. a bucket with a handle), be sure to use the other hand for support while you come to a standing position).

The Straight Leg Lift

This lift is only used when bending of the knees and hips is limited, and you cannot get close to the load. Special care must be exercised when using this lifting method to prevent aggravation of your back condition.

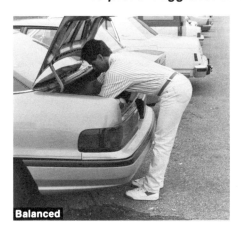
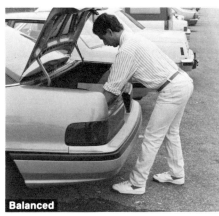
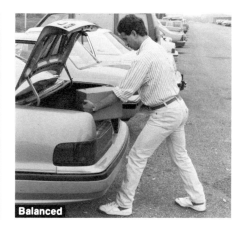

Your lower back must be kept in a balanced position and the forward bending movement must take place at the hips, not the back. Position yourself as close as possible to the load. Keep your back in a balanced position and your head up. Use your body weight and momentum to move the load, and keep the load supported (ie; on the lip of the trunk) as much as possible. *Because of the distance of the load from your body, and the increased stress that can be generated if performed incorrectly, this type of lift is not recommended during the acute and sub-acute stage.*

Summary

The main points of this manual are:

1. **Keep your back in a balanced position.**

2. **Plan your movements ahead of time.**

3. **Ask for assistance when appropriate.**

4. **Do not remain in one position for extended periods of time.**

5. **Maintain a wide stable base while standing and lifting.**

6. **Pivot your feet, don't twist your back.**

7. **Keep your stomach muscles firm while lifting and performing daily activities.**

8. **Keep items close to your body when lifting or carrying.**

9. **Lift with your legs, not your back.**

10. **When in doubt — ask your therapist or doctor.**

Your doctor or therapist may give you additional information as well as exercises to do at home. It is very important that you follow their recommendations carefully. It is also important for you to remember that *remaining inactive and being overly cautious can cause as many (or more) problems than being overly active.* This balance of rest and activity is best achieved by working closely with your doctor or therapist.

Remember that the techniques which can help you cope with your back pain are the same techniques that can prevent a recurrence of your symptoms.

Final Words

As long as you are following the principles presented in this manual, and following the instructions of your doctor and therapist, you will achieve a good balance between safe activity and rest. You have been presented with a great deal of information. You will not be able to incorporate all of these new patterns and ideas into your daily life without practice. ***What is practiced today can become habit tomorrow.***

Additional Notes

WCC 11/96